Testosterone Tales

The Robot and *I*—A New-Normal

A marginally whimsical look at what every man and the people who love them need to know when Testosterone (Androgen) deprivation is prescribed as therapy.

Harry O. Ames

Cover art and illustrations by Louise Morgan

Dedication

This book is dedicated to all of the wonderful men and women in local community medical services and those working hard throughout the United States in research laboratories and specialty hospitals to defeat cancers of all kinds.

I am alive because of the Researchers, Doctors, Nurses and other personnel who have dedicated their lives to finding new ways of extending lives and the quality of life for prostate cancer patients.

I wish particularly to thank the staff and founders of the Huntsman Cancer Institute in Salt Lake City, Utah, for providing a safe haven in my own times of medical and psychological need.

Susan, my wife of 54 years, has been my life support system for the last 22 years during which, largely to her, I've been able to live a happy and fulfilling life after being diagnosed with aggressive prostate cancer at age 52. She and our four sons and daughter have made all the difference in my motivation to "Do what the doctor says."

There are many *unsung* heroes in the fight against prostate cancer. Those are the men who are no longer with us, but whose own battles with prostate cancer have provided new information for researchers to add to the deep well of knowledge about the disease.

Disclaimer

I am a rocket scientist, not a cancer doctor or psychiatrist or psychologist. I have limited knowledge of anything medical. Your doctors, on the other hand, are not rocket scientists, but are the people who can keep you alive and living well. Listen to them. However, don't depend upon their advice if you need to launch a rocket to the moon or the planets.

I've written this booklet for the sole purpose of using my best layman's language as a surviving prostate cancer patient to communicate my view of the realities of what happens to your body and mind when you are deprived of testosterone for any reason.

This booklet would have been of great help to me had it been handed to me the first time my doctor spoke with me about testosterone deprivation. As skilled as my doctors have been in treating my metastasized prostate cancer, after they explained T-deprivation, I was left with many questions. I then turned to the internet for help. There, the technical lingo and the mix of "Oh poor me's" and "I've never felt betters" left me wandering in a fog. That was not what I needed for my already panicked and confused mind.

I've written this based upon my own experience. I hope what you read here will help you come to the conclusion, as I have, that accepting T-deprivation as a temporary or long term therapy is well worth it. It is not to be feared; life is worth living—even in that new normal.

Please let your spouse, partner or support group read this booklet. They need to understand in simple terms what you are going through. They need to be able to appreciate the courage you have to live a long and satisfying life in spite of this medical challenge.

Contents:

Preface

Oops! For us men, that is the word you never want to hear when you are having your annual physical at the doctor's office, especially when you're bent over the examining table with your pants around your knees as he conducts the dreaded DRE. I know. I know. If you

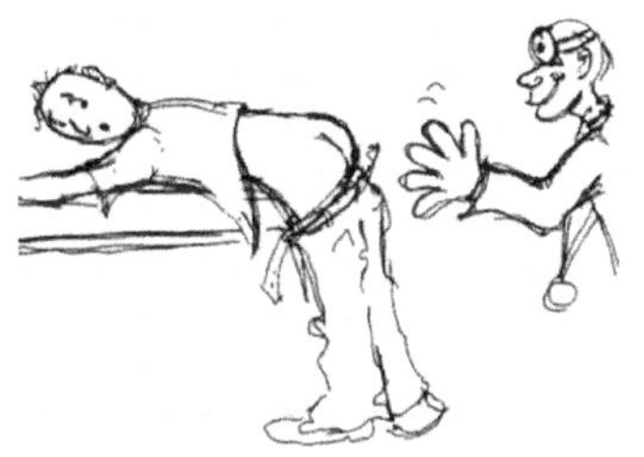

are a woman right now, you are thinking, "Oh, fine! This is nothing that I need to read about." Well, ladies, you are wrong, so be patient and read on as this information is for guys *and* the people who love them.

The "Oops" I heard in the doc's office a couple of decades ago was the discovery of prostate cancer.   "Oops" changed my world forever in some uncomfortable ways but also in many good ways.

I am currently living a *new-normal* life after three life-saving and life-extending medical interventions. Because my cancer has metastasized to a few places in my bones, the docs prescribed deployment of the gold-standard weapon against the nasty little prostate cancer cells—long term testosterone deprivation, also called androgen deprivation. In some cases and phases of prostate cancer, T-deprivation may be used for short term treatment of non-metastasized cancer cells.

T-deprivation consists of the temporary shutdown of two testosterone factories; primarily the testes, and secondarily the adrenal gland. I say "temporary" because the shutdown is induced by two drugs, Lupron and Bicalutimide. One stops the testes from working and has to be injected about every three months; the other drug temporarily shuts down the final 20% of the T production from the adrenal gland. The end result is that as long as I get those two drugs, I am T-free. Using the shots and pills is much less drastic than permanent surgical methods for stopping long term T production. I have the option at any time to stop the shot and pill. If I did, my T would return and I would be confronted with the high probability of waking up the cancer cells, and that creates a higher risk of sudden and potentially deadly growth and spread of the cancer.

I'm only one of millions of men in this country surviving physically and psychologically day-to-day and year-to-year without that most precious drop of male chemistry. Some are T challenged due to aging and some due to accident or other diseases or forms of cancer.   But many, if not most, are due to elective T deprivation for treatment of prostate cancer. Most—after a period of initial adjustment—get along fine without T and can live long and happy lives. Some let the situation ruin them.

This booklet focuses upon my own psychological and physiological experience with T deprivation due to metastasized prostate cancer. However, my layman's research validates that the effects are very common without regard to the cause for the loss of the testosterone.

T deprivation to control metastasized prostate cancer is not a cure and works for a period of time that is bounded by a complicated statistical data set that your doctors will or have explained to you.

It seems there are several classes of prostate cancer cells. I'll title them: weak, average, potent and Arnold Schwarzenegger. The Arnolds and perhaps to some degree the weaker types can all—even with T deprivation—mutate over time and grow in spite of being T starved. Though T deprivation is not a cure, it is the most common standard-of-care delaying tactic at this time. However, there are many marvelous prostate cancer treatment and intervention trials occurring across the nation that are promising to significantly delay that *awakening* phenomenon and to extend life.

I hope Testosterone Tales helps you or a loved one better deal with the powerful physiological and psychological effects of the complete loss of testosterone whether temporary or permanent.

Harry O. Ames

Chapter One

The Biological Robot and *I*

My career spans 40 years working with electrical, chemical and mechanical systems designed to go places and do things that humans simply can't: namely, to explore our wondrous solar system and the cosmos. As a child, I was fascinated with the concept of robots and shooting one into space. I figured that would be much safer than attempting to send myself off on a rocket. I built many from cigar boxes, Quaker Oats boxes, and from my favorite toy of all—my Erector Set. None of my robots lived up to my expectations nor would anyone volunteer to launch one into space. My fifth-grade teacher really let me down when he told me that he didn't know how to make a rocket.

Meanwhile, I spent many hours pondering my own body, and at a very young age I concluded that it was a fantastic biological robot in which I resided and that I could control. That initial childlike sense of my sentient self being a resident of the robot matured over the years and has helped guide me through difficult and challenging times in my 22 years walking with prostate cancer. So, to help me pass along some information that I hope will be of value to you, I've chosen to use the robot and *I* as literary tools.

Generally, I will be using the italicized capital *I* (i) to represent the conscious *you* and the word "robot" to represent the body and the *instinctive* functions it performs.

I is inside the robot, looking out on the world and has limited ability to change the way the robot processes data because it is controlled by an instinctual central processing unit which is heavily influenced by testosterone. The T grows hair and creates body odor and pheromones and fight or flight actions. It fuels the sex drive furnace and provides external indications of what *I* is feeling: anger or happiness sadness and joy.

Much of the time, *I* happily goes along for the ride, but there are many occasions when *I* is confronted with the less refined influences of the robot's T and must choose one of two actions.

1. Put the robot on autopilot and go with what the sensors are picking up—*she's sexy, he's challenging my turf, need to compete, gotta procreate, listen to that engine, what a cool new tool.*

OR:

2. Put the robot on manual control and make the robot do what it is told.

These pesky robots we inhabit instinctively procreate given the opportunity. They protect their world against intruders and threats to their robotish functions. They don't, by programming, do bad or get mad or strike out at some turf challenging brute or force sex on a female who doesn't want it. But, with the drug testosterone flowing through the system and left on its own without the influence of *I*, instinct can jump off the track and bad stuff can happen.

The robot doesn't easily give up its instinctual ways but take away the robot's T and it becomes a more compliant machine over which *I* has more control.

Chapter Two

The Robot Rebels

The post pubescent robot smoothly and quickly settles into its world of hairy armpits and BO. Its lust after the female figure and need for manly pursuits become its best friends.   Then one day the robot is diagnosed with some malfunction and the doctor tells it, "You've got prostate cancer and I'm gonna take away your T."

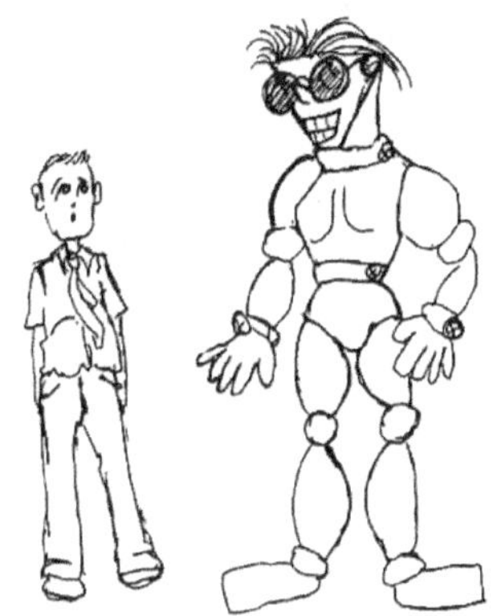

Those dreaded words set the robot's heart pounding and its central processor shoots adrenaline everywhere and the fight or flight sequence kicks in. The robot sets its facial expression to read, "What the heck did you just say, Doc?" The doctor will go into all the reasons that it is okay but that you may die if he doesn't take away the T. At least, that is what the robot hears.

Fortunately, doctors, hoping to reach past the instinctive reactions of the robot, delve more deeply in order to reach the more sensible passenger, *I*. They explain that death isn't imminent and that T deprivation is a powerful and life extending therapy. The soothing voice of the Docs gives *I* a chance to get hold of the robot's adrenaline valve and back off the flow. That gives *I* some time to ponder the whole situation without having to fight robotish sensory overload.

I's first thought is that when you are old enough to be at high risk for a disease like prostate cancer, the doctors all appear to be twelve years old and are themselves full of T and having a good time with it. You doubt that they have any firsthand knowledge about how being without it may feel.

The person best qualified to write this small booklet would be a Urological Oncologist who is in his 70's and has been through many years without T. But I've looked and haven't found one. So, I'm here doing my best, having only achieved C's in biology in high school—though I did excel at frog dissection.

For the real cellular level stuff, you need to listen to the doctors, not an exceptionally good frog dissector.

Chapter Three

The Man in Black

A few years ago I was sitting in a chair while an apprentice phlebotomist was trying unsuccessfully to find a vein in my arm from which to suck some blood. Across from me in another chair and also undergoing blood tests was a fellow who could have been Johnny Cash's younger brother. He was pale and obviously sick and had a lonely look about him. I was glad for the distraction because I don't do well with needles being wielded by a junior phlebotomist, tongue wagging enthusiastically as she pokes away at my veins.

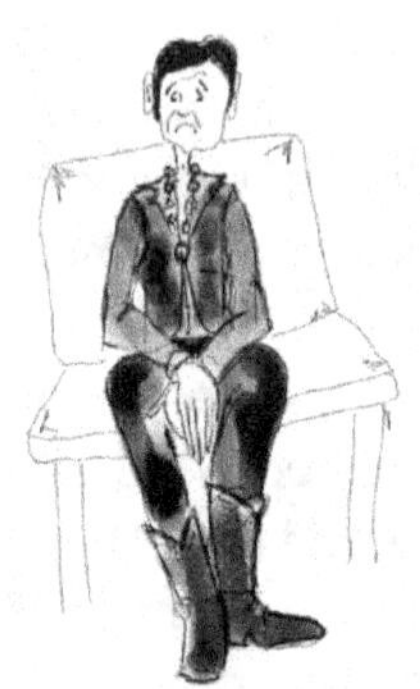

This very pale faced gentleman was all decked out in black snake-hide cowboy boots, black jeans, mostly unbuttoned black shirt with several gold chains around his neck, and a black leather vest. His hair was dyed black, and I mean the blackest black. I judged him to be 55 to 60 years old. His back story as best I could determine was that he had no current family, at least none who were of the sympathetic-caretaker mindset. He was alone with metastasized prostate cancer and was on the standard-of-care treatment like me.

The Man in Black's robot was fighting a mighty fight for its masculinity and I admired his robot for that. I could tell by looking into his eyes that his *I* was struggling and close to giving up.

For many men, perhaps most men, much of their life is built around physical manifestations of manliness to prove that they are doing manly things and thinking manly thoughts. I'm pretty sure the man in black had *done it all* over the years and that the thought of it all being gone, was taking an emotional toll. I felt very bad for the Man in Black.

There is a relatively high rate of suicide among men who have lost their testosterone, including some high profile people in the arts and sports. Many of those men experienced fame because of their super manliness and the new-normal of life without T was unacceptable.   Their robotish element won the day, because *I* declared defeat rather than force the robot to face the enemy.

It is a sad state of affairs when men choose death either by not treating their disease or through suicide, or to sit around in grumpy silence for the balance of their lives just because of the loss of their testosterone. Yes, it is a difficult psychological challenge and I'm hoping that my words will encourage and help men like the Man in Black, a once manly man, a superman, a terrific guy, "A man that all women want, but know they can never truly possess." (That approximate quote is from one of my all time favorite lines by Clive Cussler about his hero, the indisputably manliest man ever, Dirk Pitt).

Another great line comes from the fictional character, Detective Harold Oliver, a once highly paid detective who is now on hard times as he bemoans—while reflecting on his image in a mirror: "Gone were the buns of steel, the jet black hair and mustache, and the glitter of perfect bleached teeth. There were no beautiful women by my side. Instead, looking back at me was a fifty five year old, six-foot tall body with a pot belly, thinning gray hair, bloodshot eyes, wrinkles and a face full of physical and emotional scars. My outlook and every part of my body were saggy, including my shadow."

There's not enough Lupron or Bicalutimide in the world to reduce Dirk Pit's testosterone, so he would never experience Harold Oliver's emotions. On the other hand, the emotions expressed by Harold Oliver are reflective of the feelings that I've occasionally experienced during my walk down the T free road.

Chapter Four

In Search of *I*

As stated before, we are two entities in one space: the robot and *I*. The robot is biological and functions principally by instinct stored in the brain. *I* happily spends much of its time as a passenger. Aside from general guidance of the contraption, *I* is fairly comfortable letting instinct run the show. *I* frequently naps during the good times but can, when necessary, take control of the robot. *I* excels when logic and kindness and love and reason are at stake.

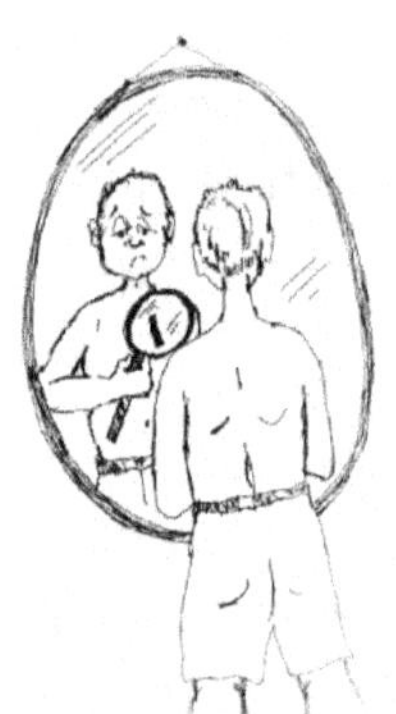

Some have observed that humans behave as though there is a good angel on one shoulder and a trouble maker on the other. The good angel is *I* and the trouble maker is likely to be the robot's instinctual programming.

Teasing-out the good angel is difficult for someone who has spent a long life enjoying the benefits and pleasures of letting the robot follow its programming, thereby providing the ready excuse in times of mischief that "The robot made me do it." So, when the T is gone and the side effects of the loss of T come into play, *I* must be fully awakened and take more control of the robot or all may be lost.

A personal note: The search for my *I* began 22 years ago. I was coasting along with my robot generally on autopilot when my wife suggested that I should go have a long overdue physical. I went to my local practitioner and he did all of the disgusting stuff, checking for hernias and the like. Then it came time for the Digital Rectal Exam (DRE). This goes beyond disgusting, but suffice it to say that it is uncomfortable at many manly levels.

 I was bent over the examination table, pants down, and feeling very undignified when from behind me I heard the word, OOPS! Not really shouted in all caps like I've shown, but that is the way my robot heard it. I immediately asked the Doc, "What do you mean, oops?" He told me that one side of my prostate was firm and that was an indication of something worth further testing. Blood was drawn, and a few days later, the report came in that my prostate specific antigen (PSA) was at

3.5. The doc told me that for a 52 year old guy, it was higher than it should be.

My next visit was with a urologist who did a water-boarding-like thing called a needle biopsy. Being water-boarded is child's play compared to the needle biopsy of the prostate. I quickly confessed everything I could think of and even made up some stuff just to have him stop with the needle.

Up to that point in time my robot and *I* had carried on a pretty balanced relationship. We'd never had any major battles—maybe one or two during the early years, but generally we had a good understanding of who controlled what. But when the biopsy results came in as prostate cancer, the robot got really crazy and the adrenaline flowed and it ran around and bounced off the living room walls. *I* struggled to take control.

Being computer savvy, *I* turned to the "best possible medical resource," the internet. After all, if it is on the internet, it must be true. Scary words like mortality and morbidity popped onto the computer display causing *I* to have to keep one foot on the head of the robot while reading about the the treatment options. When the robot heard about a thing called RPT (Radical Prostatectomy), *I* felt control over the robot slipping away as the side effects of treatment, real and potential, spilled from the computer screen. *I* was pretty sure that the robot and the computer were in cahoots to create a miserable night's sleep.

I read that the famous general, Norman Schwarzkopf, (a man with whom my military son had mingled during the freeing of Kuwait, in the 90's), had opted for the RPT. *I* figured if it was good enough for the general, a real man's man, it was good enough for *I* and the robot.

The surgery was tough and was done old-school before surgical robots and three little slits in your groin. It was the old fashioned—Let's split this guy open from his belly button to his nether parts and yank out that old rotten prostate—type of surgery. The post-surgery folks microscopically inspected the cells at the cutting edges of the now orphaned prostate and reported that no nasty cells had gotten out and all would be well. There was other good news for the robot, one of a redundant pair of happy nerves were left to allow the robot to carry on one of its favorite pastimes.

Years passed and other than for some manageable side effects, *I* was feeling pretty good about the future. The robot settled comfortably into its new physiological state and in general, life was good.

Chapter Five

Say What?

After many years of undetectable PSA, seven to be exact, and having annual PSA tests, a local practitioner told *I* that the robot's PSA was no longer in the undetectable zone. The PSA was moving up and would need frequent monitoring to see how

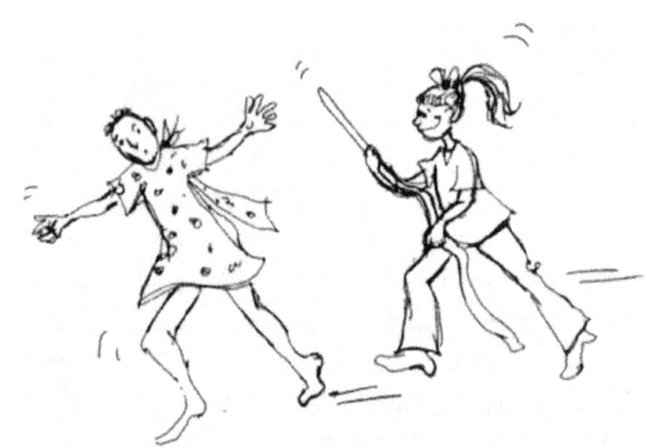

fast it was moving. Upon hearing that news and an initial bout with the robot fighting for more control, *I* was able to settle things back down a bit as the Doc gave assurances that death was not right around the corner.

A new, 16-year-old Doc suggested that the robot and *I* should trot down to the local radiation center and get the pelvic area radiated. However, an old wise friend suggested that when it comes to cancer and a man's plumbing that a specialist at a cancer research hospital should be consulted. That was done, and the specialist explained that radiation wasn't wise yet as there was nothing to indicate exactly where to target the cells that were playing tag with each other and that more waiting and watching was in order.

Then one day, the robot reported to *I* that it was not happy with the peeing process; it was a little painful. *I* took the robot to the local urologist who said he'd, "take a look." He didn't tell *I* *how* he'd take a look.

The urologist called Missy into his office and said, "Missy, please take this robot to the cystoscopy room." Missy was a very nice 11-year-old girl and while telling *I* all about her new Shitzu puppy, she led the robot to the room. *I* didn't have a smart phone to consult on every single trivial issue in those days. Not knowing what the word cystoscopy meant was troubling. Once in the room, Missy told *I* to go behind a screen and change into a hospital gown—the kind with a slit down the back that you can never actually get to cover the butt. Afterwards and expecting to find the urologist, instead, Missy was still there smiling and holding a really large syringe. She said, "Lie back and relax."

Can any manly old man relax when an 11-year-old girl is holding a big syringe full of something and she is moving in on Mr. Happy?   The robot, in complete collusion with *I,* closed its eyes and tried to pretend that Missy was actually an 80-year-old senior nurse by the name of Gertie. It was a failed mission and didn't dull the pain of having a couple quarts of Novocain going into the plumbing—really fast. Urologists who are only 16-years-old, and their 11-year-old nurses don't understand that fitting tubing with an outside diameter of a couple of inches into a receptacle that is only as big as a coffee stir-stick is not a good thing.

The doctor came in and Missy left the room with a chuckle and an evil grin on her face. Then and only then did the robot scream like a man who'd just had his nether parts invaded by one of those worms from the movie, Dune. Just as the Novocain was kicking in, the Doc came at the robot with a long tube thingy with a camera on the end and stuffed it in like Santa going down the chimney.

"Wow, what is that?" That is the second worst thing for a doctor to say to a man with a camera run up Mr. Happy.

The "that" turned out to be a pickle sized tumor that was rooted right at the old 1997 incision line when the RPT was performed. The urological oncologist took a biopsy and confirmed that the tumor was prostate cancer tissue. He took the results to the hospital tumor board where it was decided that the tumor would be surgically reduced in size after which the site would be radiated. To assure success, there was a three month round of T deprivation to allow the tissue left after the surgery to shrink a bunch more. Then there were 45 doses of radiation on the tumor to take place over a period of 45 week days so the docs could take the weekends off for video gaming or maybe some skate boarding.

Chapter Six

T or no T? That is the Question

All of the doctors on the tumor board appeared to be teenagers and had never been without T, but they had certificates on their walls and drove cool cars, so *I* decided that since it was only temporary—a fact which helped keep the robot in check—to accept the treatment; to let the Lupron be injected to temporarily put the testes to sleep and to start taking daily Bicalutimide, the drug that shuts down the adrenal glands production of T. *I*, being the intellectual part of the robot function, accepted the shots and pills philosophically, because after all, they were temporary. *I* and the robot went home arm in arm to see what would happen.

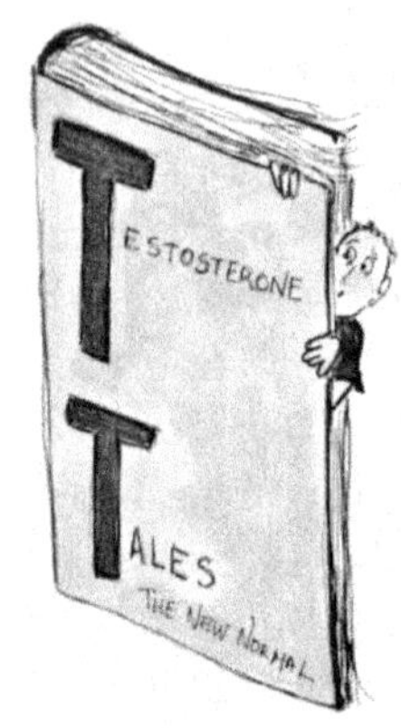

Friends teased *I* about turning into a girl and how the robots voice would move from base to soprano and other things that *I* didn't think were all that funny. But, being a manly man and focusing on the word *temporary*, *I* guffawed along with them. Meanwhile, *I* was becoming less philosophical and more worried. So, yet again, *I* resorted to the internet and didn't like what was found there.

The side effects of T deprivation were pretty obvious within a few weeks as the robot started having hot flashes every hour. In the light of day, they were mildly entertaining to *I* but at night the robot was throwing covers off and then on with a frequency that moved it out of the master bedroom so the robot's poor wife could get some sleep. Of course, *I* was losing sleep too, but—thanks to retirement—was able to hit the napping chair anytime the need came along.

The other major side effects kicked in within a month: reduced energy, waning sex drive, appetite changes and the lack of desire to get off of the couch and do something useful. The robotish aspect of the brain lost some of its sharpness and *I* started having trouble with attention span. But, the good news was that this was just temporary until the radiation was over and the tumor was dead. Being a manly man, *I* could handle the inconvenience just fine.

As the three month Lupron shot was in full effect, *I* experienced entry into a more creative state of thought. *I* was more interested in finishing writing a book that had been ignored for years. *I* began writing little essays about life and living and was enjoying travel more as it was centered on what *I* was seeing. Normally *I*'s travel was driven by robotish romantic notions, not by what might be learned.

It took another three months for all the affects of the T deprivation to wear off after the radiation and *I* became very happy until months later when the PSA was back and a bone scan showed some metastasis to the bones.

The Doctors told *I* that the metastasized cancer would be best treated with T deprivation for many years into the future. In spite of *I* being unhappy and, after a mighty struggle with the robot, *I* resolved to fight a good fight, man-up, and adapt to the new-normal.

Chapter Seven

The Only Place to Go is Up

Maslow was able to achieve fame in psychology circles by figuring out that if people can't breathe they'll die. He calls his major discovery the Pyramid of Human Needs. The bottom of the pyramid contained the most important, air—a no brainer. The top is called, "Self Actualization Needs

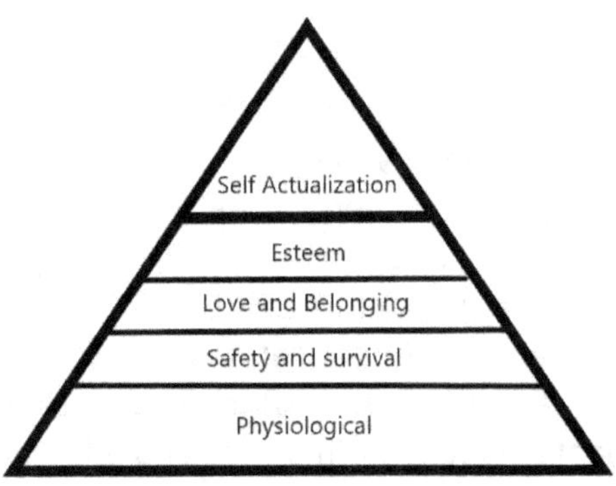

- realizing personal potential, self-fulfillment, seeking personal growth and peak experiences." (We'll stick with self actualization to shorten things up a bit).

The bottom two layers of the pyramid belong to the robot, the next three are shared decreasingly with *I*, but the top layer is *I*'s exclusive domain.

The robot's ability to function on the lower levels is instinctual, and it is very happy hanging out in those areas. It is comfortable and self centered when it comes to breathing, eating, being safe, making love and satisfying its ego. It cares very little for Self Actualization because it doesn't know it exists. In the T fueled normal, *I* rarely gets above the smog of the lower levels because it is so busy trying to keep the lid on the robot's natural and occasionally errant ways.

The primary cause of tension between *I* and the robot is a result of T. If the T is removed, the robot becomes less combative and that frees up some time for *I* to use exploring Self Actualization. *I* is free to hang out there as long and as often as it pleases without constantly monitoring the robot.

The robot doesn't know it's been T deprived. It doesn't know it feels any different, the sensors are simply reporting new things to the central processing brain and the instinctual programs in the brain default to a new normal of daily operations. It's kind of like lobsters that don't know if the water is cold or if it is hot. (I've often wondered which scientist actually spoke with a lobster while the heat was being turned up).

Chapter Eight

The reality of the T-free world

One must do without T for a good while before being able to fully understand the nuances of existence in that state. It is likely that your doctor is a young fellow, full of T, who hasn't volunteered for any T deprivation studies on his own body. Relative to the affects of T deprivation, a doctor can be like a flight-simulator gamer who understands all of the rules of flight and aerodynamics but has never flown a real airplane and he, while on the ground, is trying to talk you through your first landing while you, a non-pilot, are alone in an actual airplane.

So, for those who are experiencing or are about to experience the T-free life over the long term, there are some things you need to know right away. The trick is that you can now choose what life is and what it will be. To help you choose to prosper rather than despair in the new-normal, you need to know that you remain a man, a good man having manly thoughts and dreams. You aren't going to become feminine or anything close.

Nevertheless, because you will be spending much more time in the self-actualized part of Maslow's pyramid of human needs, those manly thoughts and dreams will turn more to the intellectual and to a new priority of what is important in life. You won't need to waste so much time and energy managing the pesky nature of a fully T fueled robot. You can still appreciate the beautiful things in the world including the female form and a well turned out muscle car restoration and sunrises and sunsets. The welfare of friends and neighbors and loved ones may become more central to your thoughts and actions.

On the other hand, T-lessness has compromised the robot's instinctive processing in ways that can't be emotionally or physically ignored by *I* or by the people who are close in *I*'s world. You and your support team of loved ones and friends can't do much to mitigate the new-normal physiology of the robot, but there are things you and they can do to minimize and even neutralize the impact upon your quality of life.

Ultimately, from one year to many years down the road it is possible that you will visit with your doctor and he or she will tell you that the cancer cells have beaten the T starvation and are now back in business. Exactly when that may happen can only be as exact as a huge volume of outcome-statistics can predict. In other words, you and others in similar circumstances aren't necessarily on the same ship due to differences in age, physical make-up and heredity.   The average numbers for progress of the disease are only that—average. If we dwell on average we are wasting our time and opportunities for a great life.

So, plan on living many years in the new-normal and you can make a great go of it. With evolving new treatments and promising new medical trials for prostate cancer it is becoming more likely that some other age or time related illness or accident may be the thing that wraps up your time on earth.

A personal note: My docs are adamant that I continue consultations with my primary care physician to make sure that my heart and overall body health remains in good condition.

The bottom line is that if you choose—after a short period of mourning—you can become as happy and fulfilled a person as you were in your prior T fueled state of the old-normal.

Chapter Nine

Sex Isn't All It's Cracked Up to Be?
You must be wrong!

Believe the doctor when he says sex drive will go away. From a fully T packed man's point of view this sounds like something absolutely horrible to even contemplate. And it is horrible to contemplate but not horrible to experience. The reason is, like the aforementioned lobster in the cooking pot, when the T is gone, the robot 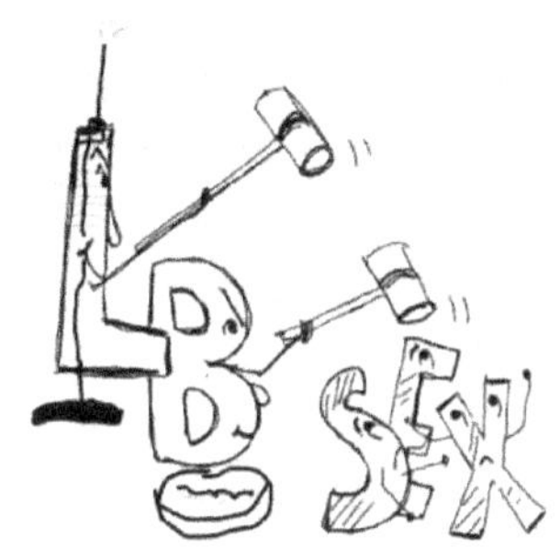 doesn't know it. It goes on about its business, adjusting systems to sustain life without T. *I* on the other hand has powerful memories of the joys of intimacy and in that regard isn't quite as adaptable as the robot

T deprivation may remove the robot's instinctive sex drive, but *I* is given the opportunity to see that true love and respect for another human being can be as emotionally fulfilling as the act of sex. Sex was the robot's domain. Love is *I*'s domain and in the self actualized state a new kind of love and intimacy can unfold in amazing and completely fulfilling ways.

Personal note: I still get great joy looking upon my cute spouse, and I definitely admire pretty ladies who cross my path day to day. In my world, men are still disgusting creations and looking at them is much like looking at road-kill. On the other hand, ladies of all ages please my eyes in much the same way as stunning sunsets, beautiful flowers or a nicely restored American muscle-car or British sports car of the 40's and 50's. Now, when I'm with my wife, I more fully appreciate the amazing creature that she is. My robot's eyes and emotions have been instinctively driven for decades by the blue eyes and the blond hair and the shapely figure of the woman I've chased around the bedroom. I don't exactly chase her around the bedroom anymore and that's okay with her and me. Without the robot's testosterone fog in place, the sense of love and completeness and bond with my spouse is now as great as or even greater than it has ever been. It has become a priceless gem that makes life worth living in the new-normal.

When I was told about the T-free side effects by the doctors, I expected that when the sex drive decrease began that I would have a sensation like stepping in from the cold into the heat or stepping out of the heat into the cold. I expected to have a noticeable loss of something. That was not the case. Sex and all its trappings simply began to disappear from my lexicon of potential activities. It was so gradual that I took no notice. I expected to mourn the loss of my sex drive as though I'd lost an arm or my eyesight. Other than pleasant memories of specific classes of events associated with that kind of intimacy there is nothing in the loss of sex drive that was dramatic enough—strangely— to even know it was gone.

It is possible that some men have built their sense of existence around sex drive. If those individuals have such a short list of life experiences, perhaps there could be a clear and undeniable sense of loss. In that case, *I* has much to do to redefine the future. The people who have such a man within their circles of concern also have much to do to help show that man a new life path and to accompany him along it.

Chapter Ten

Come on, Dude, Get off the Couch!

When the robot runs out of T, it is much like a sludged up automobile engine that is hard starting and uncooperative. Unlike the inanimate automobile engine, it simply doesn't want to be bothered by someone trying to clean it up and get it going. In fact, the robot can get 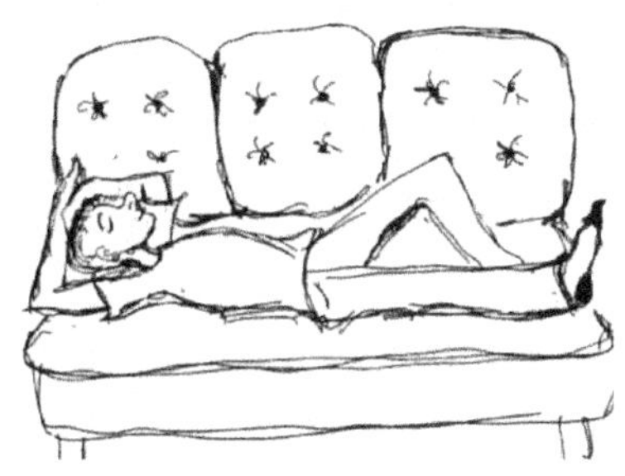 a little resentful, particularly if an entity other than *I*—perhaps a well intended loved one or friend—is trying to get the thing rolling.

The motivation issue is very important for those in the support circle to understand. *I* must also understand that the people closest to us have been used to seeing the robot cutting down the trees, carrying out the garbage, cleaning the garage, pursuing a career or jogging and climbing mountains. It can be a shock for those most familiar with the once T-fueled creature to see it sitting on the couch with a pleasant look on its face, staring off into the distance at nothing in particular, when there is so much to be done.

In regards to decreased motivation, the robot and *I* share common ground. *I* is somewhat content with couch-sitting. *I* greatly appreciates the opportunity to ponder life, the universe, and everything and drift back and forth between what has been and what is now and what may be—unhindered by a T-fueled robot. It takes an important person in *I*'s life to break through that dull eyed self realization state so loved by Maslow. Left alone, *I* and the robot will ignore the cobwebs and dust covering their inactivity as they slowly mummify there on the couch.

Sadly, that is often the case with T deprived men who have no support person or group. And that state of inactive limbo may have an unpleasant ending.

For those who are lucky enough to have a support person or group, here are some thoughts for them:

- Even though it is a fun thing to do, often brought on by the T-less person's own comments, never—and I mean never— refer to his health issue in terms such as, "Well, you might sound good as a soprano." or, "You cry so easily these days." or, "Just think, now you can enjoy all of those chick flicks that your wife likes to see." There is nothing funny about the T-less condition. Not even if the T-less guy tries to make a joke out of it. He most often is hurting at some level inside and tries to cover the hurt by joking about himself. Remember, people, he is still a man but feels like a man with an illness. You wouldn't joke about someone who lost an eye or a leg or a still born baby. Prostate cancer-standard-of-care can create the same degree of mourning for the loss of what was or could have been as any other serious personal loss or illness.

- Understand that the chemically altered robot that you've enjoyed for years doesn't respond to what would have been normal motivations to get going. Promises of excitement, adventure, sex, thrills and spills won't work very well. No matter how much it is prodded, the robot is no longer what it was and it is doing what latent natural programming does when the fuel system is altered. *I* has the only connections that might get the robot off of the couch. What interests and motivates *I*—which is now the more dominant force in the whole bipedal package—is more conversation on a much wider variety of topics than the support team is used to. His preoccupation with sports, politics, guns, fishing, new lawn mowers, save the whale, sky diving, mountain climbing, Al Gore, Trump—that whole class and a bunch of other similar ones don't automatically play in the self actualized realm of *I* anymore.

- More thoughtful action will be required on the part of the support team to get the T-less to find interests sufficient to inspire action. Pretty much without exception, those new interests will require a stronger intellectual component than before and that can create a difficult challenge for the support team—especially among the male elements—who are not T-less as they won't easily be able to get their arms around the condition in which they find their brother or friend or father or grandfather. It is hard to let go of the person who use to hoot and holler through family activities and who was ready for the most dangerous ski run and who loved the fastest car and could handle the heaviest bench press; the person who was at the leading edge of fun at a party or gathering; the person who was going to slay the business dragon, get rich and buy a yacht. Now he may best be served by encouraging and facilitating:

1. Good, entertainment, travel, concerts, museums, history, good music, and new mental challenges.
2. The enjoyment of association with friends and family
3. To volunteer in any of the hundreds of community or faith based opportunities to serve others.
4. Write a memoir or read classic books and study topics that prior to T-lessness were boring but that now may be interesting.
5. Go back to school in an interesting area of study, not for career reasons but to be able to enjoy enlightenment for the sake of enlightenment.
6. Make a job change if work remains a necessity. If the job in the old-normal is no longer inspiring, it may be time to make a major career adjustment.
7. Shed some old friends and associations and find some new ones who are more interested in intellectual rather than sensorial stimulation.
8. Learn to sail, fly an airplane, pan for gold, wood-carve, paint, etc. You get the picture!
9. Having a good pet and lots of attention from loved ones will motivate the T-less to find more joy in the new-normal.

Chapter Eleven

I'm so Tired, Edna.

Assuming that friends and loved ones and *I* have been successful in applying motivation therapy to the T-less, another less easily managed standard-of-care side effect comes into play. Motivation is psychological and may cause movement, but physiologically, there will be a reduction in energy and stamina.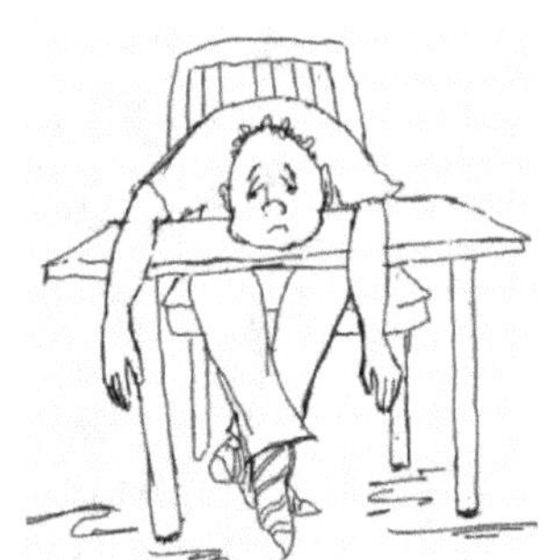

A good program of diet and exercise can minimize the effects, but the body will tire more easily.

There are many stories of the T-less guy who wins his first triathlon. That guy has some super-motivators, but for the rest of us, diving into a life style of highly disciplined exercise and diet may not be realistically attainable. It would be excellent if you can do it, so get down there on the floor and give me 25 single hand pushups, soldier! What! You don't feel like it?

Let's couple the previous section on motivation to this section on energy level. I've talked about the need to create motivations that appeal on an intellectual level. A simple example would be creating and caring for a garden. Gardening is an intellectual activity that requires physical effort. Owning a dog can be an intellectual exercise to provide care for the dog and requires the physical exertion to play with and walk the dog. I've always been fascinated with the idea of an aquarium that is a sea water aquarium; that is very intellectual and takes physical work daily to keep it operating. Photography—I mean good photography—is a very healthy and intellectual pursuit that can provide many hours of opportunity to get out and move about. Volunteerism can be an intellectual experience that is very satisfying and that will in most cases require useful physical activity.

Walking and moderate hiking in new and interesting areas close to home or far away, especially in areas that have an interesting geological or historical context, is a magnificent way to couple the intellect with physical activity.

I've said much about the need for support people to provide external stimulus to motivate and inspire the T-less, but there is an even larger responsibility for *I* to power through and move the robot to physical activity.

A personal note: My own T-less physical activities include one-mile walks over a couple of hills that push my heart into the cardio health zone. I pick a daily project around the house or on one of my cars or boats that keep me moving for at least four hours a day. I've been fortunate to have developed repair skills that serve me well on automobiles and boats and my home.   I used to be able to sustain a good long eight-hour day working on my possessions, and often longer. But now, four hours of moderate to hard physical work puts me down for rest and maybe even a nap. I can usually put in another two hours after an hour or two rest-break. Given the choice between the gym and working on my home projects, I far prefer putting in my physical exercise working on a project or walking and hiking and travel.

The T-less condition is an excellent opportunity to expand interests in areas that push the need for new physical activity—areas that the T may have blocked in the past.

Chapter Twelve

Is it just Me, or is it Warm in Here?

Truly the most irritating part of the T-less state is hot flashes. Many of us have heard a wife or mother or other female in our circle of acquaintances speak of hot flashes. As men, we chuckle and find mild entertainment in watching the ladies have hot flashes.

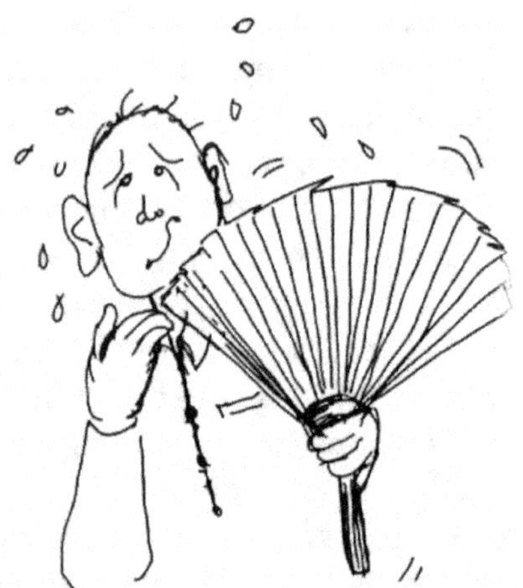

Oh, but revenge can be sweet for the ladies who have experienced hot flashes when a man they know has been deprived of his testosterone and begins to experience that weird physical phenomenon.

Hot flashes will begin relatively quickly as the Lupron and Bicalutimide start working. Hot flashes are exactly what they feel like. Suddenly and without warning your face will get hot. It isn't quite like a fever you may have experienced which is felt more throughout your body. A hot flash is very head focused. About the time you have flung off your coat or even shirt or if in bed, the blankets, you will break out into a cold sweat much like when a fever breaks if you've had a virus. It breaks out suddenly and you will be hunting a tissue or towel to dry you face.

During the minute or two of the hot flash you will feel like lying down. You may experience a sense of wanting a quick nap, but that passes very quickly. I've had many hot flashes while driving and the sense of wanting to just close the eyes and get a nap has never created a dangerous situation; especially as you come to understand the hot flash and how it specifically affects you. Some hot flash events are longer and less intense. Some are shorter and much more intense. This variation is completely unpredictable as is the frequency of occurrence of hot flashes themselves.

A personal note: The hot flashes early after my T-deprivation occurred every hour or so for 24 hours a day. It caused me to lose sleep and my moving about and throwing blankets on and off made it more comfortable for me and my wife to set up another bedroom.

Month by month over a period of two years, my hot flashes have declined in intensity and frequency, but the duration has remained about the same. I can now generally sleep through the night, though I know that I have several hot flashes while I'm asleep.

The medical folks will suggest that eventually a point comes when the hot flashes will, for all practical purposes, stop. They may be right, but two years into my T-less new normal, they still happen and though less frequent, they are an irritant.

The good news is, generally speaking, hot flash experiences vary widely from man to man and that they will be more bothersome early on and much less bothersome over time.

An additional interesting thing about hot flash events is that when I am physically active, they seem to be fewer and less intense. It may also be that that physical activity can be distracting enough that you simply are less aware that a hot flash is taking place. That is especially true on warm or hot days.

Chapter Thirteen

Why Am I crying?

I've emphasized earlier that you are still a man when deprived of testosterone. But, because you are spending more time in the top of Maslow's pyramid, your empathic qualities become magnified. You will be thinking serious thoughts about life and living and interpersonal relationships. If you have a favorite pet that dies, that event will become much more emotionally intense than what you would feel before having T-deprivation. And

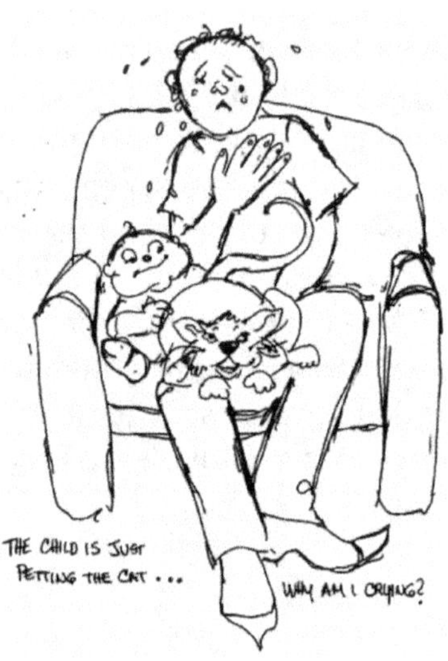

that will be even more so if you lose a loved one or if family members or friends are hurting. You will be more uplifted by great music and entertainment. Your choice in reading material and televised materials will lean much more to that which is intellectually stimulating. Don't fight that side benefit of the new-normal.

You will cry more. Yes, Mr. Manly Man, you will tear up more, so get used to it. Those tears aren't tears of weakness, but rather tears which will tell you that *I* is now in charge of the robot. The tears can be a healthy therapy for your new normal.

I will still have memories of past days and glories and activities that are no longer practical in the new normal and that can cause periods of grumpiness and a somber mood. If a support person or loved one points that out to you, it is up to you to understand and walk away from those moods. It is also important for that support person or loved one to understand that sometimes your moods are not easily dismissed. Moods, happy or sad, are to a large extent a decision and with practice you can overcome their negative effects on yourself and those around you.

Chapter Fourteen

Hey! What Happened to My Chest Hair?

Hair production on your body will slow way down over time.

A personal note: After two years, my once hairy arms and legs are still hairy, but with fine downy hair. That is true over all of my body. I've not lost my head hair, but it has thinned a bit and is somewhat unruly.

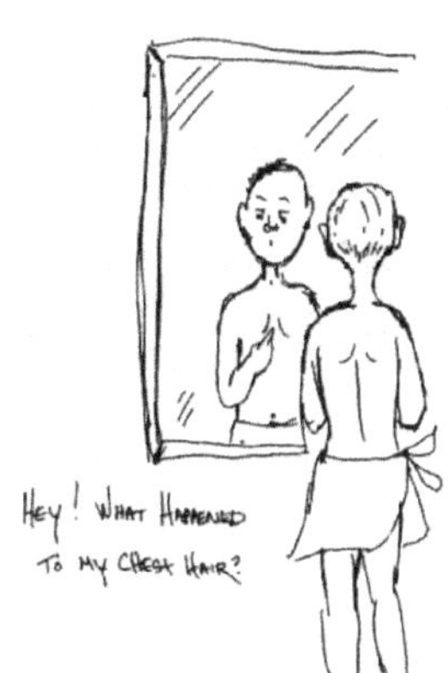

A real advantage I now have is shaving only once a week, and sometimes even once every 10 days.

Another advantage is that I used to produce a lot of body odor when physically active, challenging even the best deodorants. Now I have no body odor at all.

Maintaining muscle mass is a major challenge. I have maintained weight, but muscle mass has been replaced by some flab. For me, the flab is and will be a big challenge in the new-normal.

Final Thoughts

I've been living in the new-normal for over two years as of the date of this writing. I can honestly guarantee that the new-normal is not as much fun as the old-normal. I can also honestly guarantee, that if *I* takes control of the robot and accepts the new-normal rather than fighting it and seeks out new ways of living and experiencing life, that life is truly worth living and fighting for. You can experience a new world that was likely often ignored and out of reach during the old-normal. That world is in the top-cap of Maslow's pyramid.   Remember it?

"Self Actualization Needs:

Realizing personal potential, self-fulfillment, seeking personal growth and peak experiences"

A new world of wondrous possibilities is ahead on your journey. Wrap your arms around those possibilities and make them bow to the will of *I*.

Special Note: Many men are lucky to have spouses and loved ones in the form of children and friends who will actively seek to be their rock and strength in the new-normal. Conversely, many men, perhaps like The Man in Black, don't have such people to brace and support their journey. Your *I* needs to take every advantage of creating new and healthy and lasting relationships. Professional counseling is available and of high value. Your medical care providers can be first-responders in helping you find the support that you will need day to day that will ease your journey along the road of the new-normal.

My heart and soul are with you on your journey. Good luck, my friends.

Harry O. Ames

Here is a quick summary of my journey with prostate cancer:

1996-52 years old and diagnosed with moderately aggressive prostate cancer-PSA 3.5

January 1997-Prostatectomy-PSA soon undetectable.

2005 PSA is back but less than 1. Docs said "Not unusual to come back" and to wait and watch.

2005 thru 2012-PSA is up to 7. Docs found prostate tissue tumor at the old RPT incision site in the bladder.

Late in 2012-Docs took away the T with drugs and by Early 2013 surgically reduced the bladder tumor in preparation for local radiation. Radiation was 45 trips to hospital, one session each week day.

2013-Mid year-PSA at zero and T fully restored.

2014-Early in the year-PSA back and increasing.

2015-Late summer-Bone scans showed metastasized but tiny spots on some bones. Docs put me on permanent T deprivation. 2015-Fall-Qualified for trial drug called Palbociclib (Ibrance) that should slow the waking up of the prostate cancer cells.

2015-Publish date of this booklet-PSA undetectable.

I've tried to treat the very serious disease of prostate cancer with only a little bit of humor in a few select places in the booklet. So, as an informal appendix, I've picked a few examples of dozens of events that tickled my funny bone during my journey and still cause me to smile when I think about them.

Anecdote 1

This is just one example of many silly things that have happened working with the doctors.

I was in the urologist's office for a follow-up after the radical prostatectomy surgery. He wanted to do a digital rectal exam to check the now vacant prostate bed. I was reluctant because I hate that exam and I didn't have a prostate, but I said it was okay to do. When he came into the exam room he was accompanied by a very young and very lovely and very blonde assistant, or so I thought. He introduced her as Bamby Baumgartner. I shook her hand and she smiled pleasantly. The doctor said, "Now, Mr. Ames if you will drop your pants I'll begin the exam." I gave the doctor a patient look and said I would, but what about Ms. Baumgartner? He told me that she was finishing her medical training and was doing her post graduate rounds and was now on the urological circuit and accompanying him for a week or two. I suspected that Bamby had seen a man's bare butt many times, but it didn't make me anymore comfortable to have her there.

While the dock slapped on the rubber gloves, I dropped my pants, and turned around and leaned over the examining table. As he was hemming and hawing doing the exam, I heard the snapping sound of another pair of rubber gloves. The doc said, now Bamby, it is important for you to know what a vacant prostate bed feels like so... .

Anecdote 2

This is about friends and loved ones who are full of sympathy, but can't get their arms around what is happening to you, the cancer patient.

I have a very good friend who I've known since grade school. Our paths have crossed many times through the intervening six decades and even with a year or more between visits, we have been more like brothers than friends. He has followed my prostate cancer history with great interest and with great sympathy. About the time that I was diagnosed with metastasized cancer, I called him to fill him in on the new development. He is an accountant and expects life to move along like a tax form, so I'm careful about using any of the medical lingo that I've picked up as a cancer survivor.

I got him on the phone and said, "My cancer has progressed to the bones in a few small spots so the doctors are going to have me go on the standard-of-care which is taking all of my testosterone away." There was a very long pause and I heard him sadly shouting to his wife with tears in his voice "Gerty, they're gonna chop off Harry's balls!"

It took a full thirty minutes to settle my friend down and get him to understand that my *boys* were staying firmly in place and that I could stop the T deprivation any time I wished. You would have to know my friend and have listened in on that phone call for full humorous effect, but I include it here and maybe you can see why I couldn't stop laughing when he shouted, "Gerty!"

Anecdote 3

This is about the medical machines and the people who operate them.

During radiation for my bladder prostate tissue tumor I had to drive 180 miles round trip everyday to the cancer hospital. My wife and I did that every week day for about 50 trips which includes several of the trial runs to test positioning etc. My wife always went with me. We would get up early in the morning, have some breakfast, and I'd have my morning *cold-caffeine* in the form of a Pepsi. Understand that when I was on the radiation table, that the docs wanted some urine in the bladder, but not too much. They couldn't quite define the right amount nor how I was supposed to figure it out. So, I kept adjusting the time—from when I had my last sip of Pepsi and my last pee before leaving the house—to arrive at the radiation table with just the right amount of urine in the bladder.

However, I was often cheerily chastised by the nurses and technicians operating the big machine that my bladder was too full or not full enough, but was "adequate." Generally I came up too empty for perfection. So, one morning I slipped a small plastic container of urine looking apple juice into my coat and after gowning, I put the container into a pocket on the gown. When I lay down on the table, sure enough, the chief machine operator did an ultrasound to check the bladder contents and commented that I was a bit low. So, I said, "don't worry, I've brought extra." I reached into my gown pocket and pulled out the unlabeled little container of apple juice and quickly swallowed it. They were only momentarily horrified, but it became one of the few memorable and light hearted moments when I was on the table under the rays of the machine.

About the Author

Harry Ames lives with his wife, Susan, in Providence, Utah and is a graduate of Idaho State University and Pepperdine University.

He has five grown children and 13 grandchildren.

The bulk of his career was as a program and laboratory manager with the California Institute of Technology—Jet Propulsion Laboratory and with the Utah State University—Space Dynamics Laboratory.

Testosterone Tales is his first work of nonfiction.

Testosterone Tales is available on Amazon in soft cover or Kindle.

Harry is also the author of the currently published whimsy detective novel, titled Harold Oliver-Detective. Harold Oliver is available on Amazon in Kindle or Soft cover.

Harry Ames
PO Box 342
Providence, UT
84332

Questions or comments?

hames57@gmail.com

Phone-435 757 7695